Summary

New federal tax credits were authorized in the Patient Protection and Affordable Care Act (ACA, P.L. 111-148, as amended), to help certain individuals pay for health insurance coverage, beginning in 2014.

ACA requires "American Health Benefit Exchanges" to be established in every state by January 1, 2014, either by the state itself or by the Secretary of Health and Human Services (HHS). Exchanges will not be insurers, but will provide eligible individuals and small businesses with access to private health insurance plans. Generally, the plans offered through the exchanges will provide comprehensive coverage and meet all ACA market reforms, as applicable. One of the requirements that most exchange plans must meet is to provide a certain level of coverage generosity based on actuarial value. Each level of coverage generosity is designated according to a precious metal and corresponds to a specific actuarial value: Bronze (actuarial value of 60%), Silver (70%), Gold (80%), and Platinum (90%).

To make exchange coverage more affordable, certain individuals will receive premium assistance in the form of federal tax credits. The premium credit will be an advanceable, refundable tax credit, meaning taxpayers need not wait until the end of the tax year in order to benefit from the credit, and may claim the full credit amount even if they have little or no federal income tax liability. Although the premium credits will not be available until 2014, the illustrations provided in this report are based on current federal poverty levels, to reflect how the estimated premium credit amounts compare to current income levels.

Under ACA, the amount received in premium credits is based on income tax returns. These amounts are reconciled in the next year and can result in overpayment of premium credits if income increases, which must be repaid to the federal government. ACA limited the amount of required repayments. Since the enactment of ACA, these limits have been increased in order to raise revenues for other legislative initiatives (e.g., P.L. 111-309 and P.L. 112-9). Most recently, on June 7, 2012, the House passed H.R. 436, the Health Care Cost Reduction Act of 2012, which includes a measure that would remove all limits on repayment, making individuals fully liable for the full amount of any premium credit overpayment.

Relative affordability of health insurance premiums individuals and families might face within health insurance exchanges will likely vary from exchange to exchange based on a host of factors, including enrollees' age, the varying prices paid by plans for medical goods and services, the breadth of the provider network, the provisions regarding how out-of-network care is paid for (or not), and the use of tools by the plan to reduce health care utilization (e.g., prior authorization for certain tests). Examples provided in the **Appendix** of this report depict a range by which premiums might reasonably be expected to vary based on enrollees' age, and variation in medical costs across geographic areas, for purposes of illustration only. Actual premiums will likely vary among health insurance exchanges based on a wide range of factors other than those depicted in this report.

Contents

Figures

Tables

Appendixes

Contacts

New federal tax credits were authorized in the Patient Protection and Affordable Care Act (ACA, P.L. 111-148, as amended), to help certain individuals pay for health insurance coverage, beginning in 2014. The tax credits will go towards the cost of purchasing coverage offered through health insurance exchanges—marketplaces offering comprehensive, private health plans.

This report describes who will be eligible for the premium credits,[1] and how the credit amounts will be calculated. It also highlights key issues raised by the Internal Revenue Service (IRS) in the notice of proposed rulemaking (NPRM) on the premium credits.[2] The **Appendix** provides analysis of the concept of "affordability" as applicable to the premium credits.

Background

ACA[3] requires "American Health Benefit Exchanges" to be established in every state by January 1, 2014, either by the state itself or by the Secretary of Health and Human Services (HHS). Exchanges will not be insurers, but will provide eligible individuals and small businesses with access to private health insurance plans.[4] Generally, the plans offered through the exchanges will provide comprehensive coverage and meet all ACA market reforms, as applicable. One of the requirements that most exchange plans must meet is to provide a certain level of coverage generosity based on actuarial value.[5] Each level of coverage generosity is designated according to a precious metal and corresponds to a specific actuarial value: Bronze (actuarial value of 60%), Silver (70%), Gold (80%), and Platinum (90%).

Certain individuals who enroll in exchange coverage will be eligible for premium assistance in the form of federal tax credits. The premium credit will be an advanceable, refundable tax credit, meaning taxpayers need not wait until the end of the tax year in order to benefit from the credit (advance payments will actually go directly to the insurer),[6] and may claim the full credit amount even if they have little or no federal income tax liability.

According to the Congressional Budget Office (CBO), 29 million individuals are projected to be enrolled in exchange coverage in 2019. Of those, 19 million are projected to receive premium credits[7] (see **Figure 1**).

---

[1] Certain individuals who qualify for premium credits will also qualify for cost-sharing subsidies to help pay for deductibles, copayments, etc. The cost-sharing subsidies are outside the scope of this report.

[2] *Federal Register,* Vol. 76, No. 159, August 17, 2011.

[3] Hereinafter, "ACA" will refer to P.L. 111-148, as amended.

[4] Exchanges are designed to offer nongroup policies and small group plans. Large groups may participate in exchanges, at state option, beginning in 2017.

[5] Actuarial value is a summary measure of a plan's generosity, expressed as the percentage of medical expenses estimated to be paid by the insuer for a standard population and set of allowed charges. The higher the percentage, the more generous the coverage.

[6] §412(a)(3).

[7] CBO letter to Speaker Pelosi, ACA cost estimate, March 20, 2010, p. 9 and Table 4, http://cbo.gov/ftpdocs/113xx/doc11379/AmendReconProp.pdf'sAmendmenttoReconciliationProposal.pdf.

Figure 1. CBO: Projected Exchange Enrollment, 2019

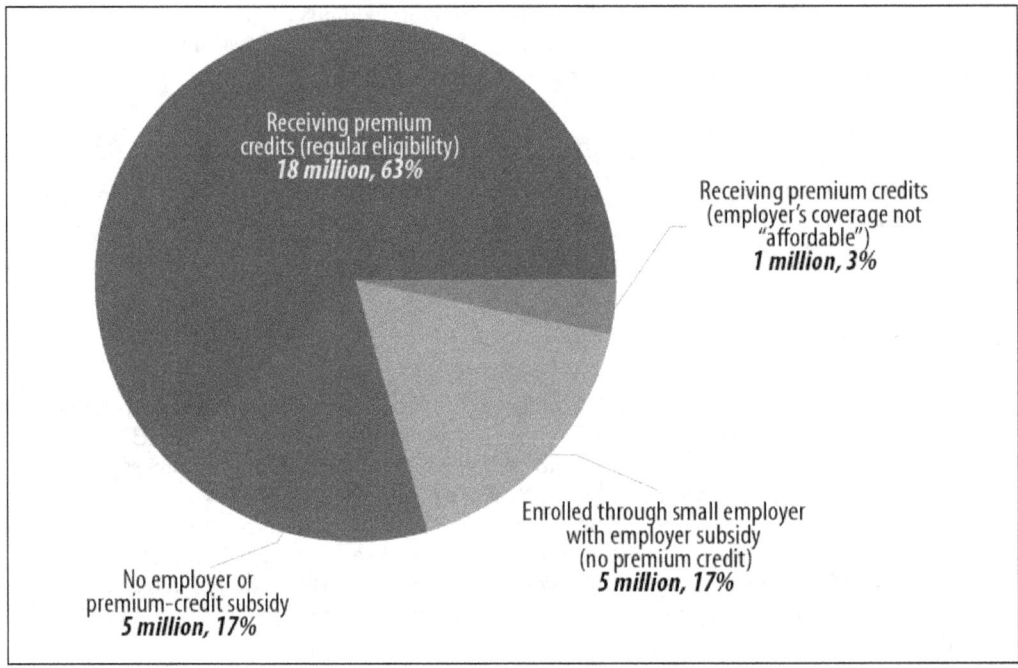

Source: CBO letter to Speaker Pelosi, ACA cost estimate, March 20, 2010, p. 9 and Table 4, http://cbo.gov/ftpdocs/113xx/doc11379/AmendReconProp.pdf.

Note: Beginning in 2014, an employer's coverage is not "affordable" when the employee's contribution toward the employer's lowest-cost self-only premiums would exceed 9.5% of household income. Employees with an employer offer of coverage may also be eligible for premium credits if the employer plan does not provide minimum value (i.e., covers less than 60% of total allowed costs). However, the CBO projection of individuals e igible for premium credits (besides meeting other eligibi ity criteria) because the employer plan would not provide minimum value was well under 1 million, and therefore not included in CBO published projections or in this figure.

As part of the ACA implementation process, the Treasury Department issued a notice of proposed rulemaking (NPRM), on the ACA premium credits in the Federal Register on August 17, 2011.[8] While the proposed rule confirmed certain eligibility and other requirements as specified in the statute, it also requested comments on various implementation issues, including flexibility with respect to the timing of eligibility (and ineligibility) for premium credits, employee and employer safe harbors, coverage of all family members in one or multiple plans, tax units with mid-year changes in family composition or filing status, and other issues. The NPRM also announced an opportunity for the public to present oral comments during a public hearing; it was held on November 17, 2011.

---

[8] "Health Insurance Premium Tax Credit," 26 CFR Part 1, *Federal Register*, Vol. 76, No. 159, August 17, 2011, available online at http://www.gpo.gov/fdsys/pkg/FR-2011-08-17/pdf/2011-20728.pdf.

Individual Eligibility for Premium Credits

ACA specifies that premium credits will be available to "applicable taxpayers" in a "coverage month" beginning in 2014.

An *applicable taxpayer* is an individual who

- is part of a tax-filing unit,
- is enrolled in an exchange plan, and
- has household income between 100% and 400% of the federal poverty level (exception described below).

A *coverage month* refers to a month in which the applicable taxpayer paid for coverage offered through an exchange, not including any month in which the taxpayer was eligible for "minimum essential coverage" with exceptions (described below).

These eligibility criteria are discussed in greater detail below.

Part of a Tax-Filing Unit

Given that the premium assistance will be provided in the form of tax credits, they will be administered through individual tax returns (although advance payments will go directly to insurers).[9] The credits can only be obtained by qualifying individuals who file federal tax returns.

Couples married at the end of the taxable year will have to file joint returns to be eligible for the credit. The NPRM includes special rules relating to the calculation of credit amounts in response to changes in filing status (e.g., taxpayers who marry or divorce during tax year), and requests comments on related operational issues (e.g., flexibility in meeting the requirement for married couples to file jointly).

Enrolled in an Exchange Plan

Premium credits will only be available to individuals enrolled in a plan offered through an exchange.[10] Individuals may enroll in a plan through their state's exchange if they are (1) residing in a state in which an exchange was established; (2) not incarcerated, except individuals in custody pending the disposition of charges; and (3) lawful residents.

Only lawful residents may obtain exchange coverage. Undocumented aliens will be prohibited from obtaining coverage through an exchange, even if they could pay the entire premium without any subsidy.[11] Because ACA prohibits undocumented aliens from obtaining exchange coverage, they will not be eligible for premium credits.

---

[9] §1412(a)(3).

[10] §1401, adding a new §36B(c)(2)(A)(i) to the Internal Revenue Code.

[11] §1312(f)(3). For more information about the treatment of noncitizens under ACA, see CRS Report R40889, *Noncitizen Eligibility and Verification Issues in the Health Care Reform Legislation.*

The NPRM clarifies the potential credit eligibility for family members of individuals who themselves may not be eligible to enroll in an exchange due to incarceration or legal status (e.g., when there is a family of four and one of the family members is incarcerated).

Household Income Is 100%-400% of Federal Poverty Level

To be eligible for premium credits, individuals must have "household income" within statutorily defined guidelines based on the federal poverty level (FPL).[12] For purposes of premium credit eligibility, household income is measured according to the current tax definition for "modified adjusted gross income" (MAGI).[13] An individual whose MAGI is at or above 100% FPL up to 400% FPL may be eligible to receive premium credits,[14] beginning in 2014.[15]

For illustrative purposes only, **Table 1** displays the income levels at 400% FPL, the amount at which individuals will *no* longer be eligible for any premium credit, if the credits were available in 2011.[16]

Table 1. Income Levels at 400% FPL, 2011

Number of Persons in Family	48 Contiguous States and DC	Alaska	Hawaii
1	$43,560	$54,400	$50,160
2	$58,840	$73,520	$67,720
3	$74,120	$92,640	$85,280
4	$89,400	$111,760	$102,840
5	$104,680	$130,880	$120,400
6	$119,960	$150,000	$137,960

[12] The FPL used for public program eligibility varies by family size and by whether the individual resides in the 48 contiguous states and the District of Columbia versus Alaska or Hawaii. See "Annual Update of the HHS Poverty Guidelines," 76 *Federal Register* 3637-3638, January 20, 2011, http://aspe.hhs.gov/poverty/11fedreg.pdf.

[13] In Section 2002(a) and Section 1401(a) of ACA, household income is defined to be MAGI in compliance with the Internal Revenue Code (IRC). With respect to the federal tax code, gross income is total income minus certain exclusions (e.g., public assistance payments, employer contributions to health insurance payments). From gross income, adjusted gross income (AGI) is calculated to reflect a number of deductions, including trade and business deductions, losses from sale of property, and alimony payments. MAGI is defined as AGI plus certain foreign earned income and tax-exempt interest. However, for premium credit eligibility purposes, the definition of MAGI will include non-taxable Social Security benefits (as amended in P.L. 112-56). For additional discussion about the use of MAGI with respect to ACA premium credits, see CRS Report R41997, *Definition of Income in ACA for Certain Medicaid Provisions and Premium Credits*.

[14] An exception is made for lawfully present aliens with income below 100% of the FPL, who are ineligible for Medicaid for the first five years that they are lawfully present. These taxpayers will be treated as though their income is exactly 100% of FPL for purposes of the premium credit.

[15] Given the interaction between the ACA's provisions on exchanges and Medicaid, most individuals with income between 100% and 133% FPL will be eligible for Medicaid, beginning in 2014. For additional information about the Medicaid provisions in the ACA, see CRS Report R41210, *Medicaid and the State Children's Health Insurance Program (CHIP) Provisions in ACA Summary and Timeline*.

[16] The FPL used for public program eligibility, the Federal Poverty Guideline, varies by family size and by whether the individual resides in the 48 contiguous states and the District of Columbia versus Alaska or Hawaii. See "Annual Update of the HHS Poverty Guidelines," 76 Federal Register 3637-3638, January 20, 2011, http://aspe.hhs.gov/poverty/11fedreg.pdf.

Number of Persons in Family	48 Contiguous States and DC	Alaska	Hawaii
7	$135,240	$169,120	$155,520
8	$150,520	$188,240	$173,080

Source: CRS computation based on "Annual Update of the HHS Poverty Guide ines," 76 Federal Register 3637-3638, January 20, 201 1, http://aspe.hhs.gov/poverty/11fedreg.pdf.

Notes: Under ACA, premium credits for eligible exchange coverage will not be available until 2014; the data in this table are for illustrative purposes only. The data are the income levels at which individuals would *not* be e igible for premium credits, if such credits were made available in 201 1. "DC" is the District of Columbia. The Federal Poverty Guidelines are updated annually for inflation.

Not Eligible for "Minimum Essential Coverage"

To be eligible for a premium credit, an individual may *not* be *eligible* for "minimum essential coverage," with exceptions (described below). ACA broadly defines minimum essential coverage to include Medicare Part A, Medicaid, the Children's Health Insurance Program (CHIP), Tricare, Tricare for Life, the veteran's health care program, the Peace Corps program, any government plan (local, state, federal) including the Federal Employees Health Benefits Program (FEHBP), any plan established by an Indian tribal government, any plan offered in the individual health insurance market, any employer-sponsored plan, any grandfathered health plan,[17] and any other coverage (such as a state high risk pool) recognized by the HHS Secretary.[18]

Exceptions to Minimum Essential Coverage Eligibility

ACA provides certain exceptions regarding eligibility for minimum essential coverage and eligibility for premium credits. An individual who is only eligible to obtain coverage through the individual (nongroup) health insurance market may be eligible to receive a premium credit. Also, an individual eligible for, but not enrolled in, an employer-sponsored plan may still be eligible for premium credits if the employer's coverage is either (1) not "affordable;" that is, the employee's premium contribution toward the employer's self-only plan would exceed 9.5% of household income;[19] or (2) does not provide "minimum value;" that is, the plan's payments cover less than 60% of total allowed costs on average.[20] As shown in **Figure 1**, of the 29 million individuals projected by CBO to be enrolled in exchange coverage in 2019, approximately 1 million are projected to be enrolled because their employer's coverage is not "affordable."[21]

---

[17] A grandfathered health plan is a group health plan or health insurance coverage (including coverage from the individual health insurance market) in which a person was enrolled on and since the date of enactment of ACA. For additional information about grandfathered plans, see CRS Report R41166, *Grandfathered Health Plans Under the Patient Protection and Affordable Care Act (ACA)*.

[18] The Treasury Department, in the NPRM on premium credits, requested comments on the transition of individuals from exchange coverage to public coverage (such as Medicaid). The comment period ended on October 31, 2011, and a public hearing was held on November 17, 2011. *Federal Register*, Vol. 76, No. 159, Aug. 17, 2011.

[19] The Treasury Department, in the NPRM on premium credits, proposed an employee safe harbor that would allow an employee to be eligible for premium credits, even if the employer plan was later determined to be affordable. The comment period ended on October 31, 2011, and a public hearing was held on November 17, 2011. *Federal Register*, Vol. 76, No. 159, Aug. 17, 2011.

[20] §1401(a), adding a new §36B(c)(2)(C) to the Internal Revenue Code.

[21] CBO letter to Speaker Pelosi, ACA cost estimate, March 20, 2010, p. 9 and Table 4, http://www.cbo.gov/ftpdocs/113xx/doc11379/Manager'sAmendmenttoReconciliationProposal.pdf.

Individual's Employer Does Not Contribute Toward Exchange Plan

Certain small employers (and in later years, potentially larger employers) may offer and contribute toward coverage through an exchange. If an individual is enrolled in an exchange through an employer who contributed toward that coverage, the individual will not be eligible for premium credits.[22]

Medicaid

Although ACA's Medicaid provisions are generally beyond the scope of this report, eligibility for Medicaid as expanded under ACA interacts with the provisions regarding premium credits for exchange coverage. From 2011 to 2013, states have the *option* to expand Medicaid to all non-elderly, non-pregnant individuals (i.e., childless adults and certain parents, except for those ineligible based on certain noncitizenship status) who are otherwise ineligible for Medicaid up to 133% FPL. Beginning in 2014, states with Medicaid programs will be *required* to extend Medicaid to these individuals.[23] In other words, the medical or family status of low-income individuals (pregnant, without children, etc.) will not matter for purposes of Medicaid eligibility. All non-elderly *citizens* (and certain *legal* aliens) with income up to 133% FPL will be eligible for Medicaid beginning in 2014. (ACA does not change noncitizens' eligibility for Medicaid.[24]) If a person who applied for premium credits in an exchange is determined to be eligible for Medicaid, the exchange must have them enrolled in Medicaid.[25]

Potential Premium Contributions and Premium Credit Calculations

The amount of the tax credit will vary from person to person: it depends on the household income of the taxpayer (and dependents), the premium for the exchange plan in which the taxpayer (and dependents) is (are) enrolled, and other factors. In certain instances, the credit amount may cover the entire premium and the taxpayer pays nothing towards the premium (see text box, scenario A). In other instances, the taxpayer may be required to pay part (or all) of the premium (see text box, scenario B).

---

[22] §1401 of ACA, adding a new §36B(c)(2)(A)(ii) to the Internal Revenue Code.

[23] ACA specifies that an income disregard in the amount of 5% FPL will be used to determine Medicaid eligibility based on MAGI; thus the effective minimum income eligibility threshold for such individuals in this new eligibility group will be 138% FPL.

[24] As under law prior to ACA, certain lawfully present aliens are eligible for full Medicaid benefits (e.g., refugees, asylees, and some legal permanent residents (LPRs) who have been here at least five years) while others are not (e.g., certain LPRs who have been here less than five years).

[25] §1311(d)(4) and §1413(a).

Calculation of Premium Credit Amounts

The premium credit amount will be the lesser of either:

(A) The cost of the exchange plan that the taxpayer (and dependents) is (are) enrolled in;

Or

(B) The excess, if any, resulting from the following formula:

The age-adjusted premium for the second lowest cost silver plan in the taxpayer's area,

Minus

The product of the taxpayer's household income and the "applicable percentage" (based on the taxpayer's household income relative to the federal poverty level).

Premium Contribution

If the premium credit amount (i.e., the lesser amount calculated above) is:

(A), then the taxpayer (and dependents) pay(s) nothing towards the premium for exchange coverage.

(B), then the individual (and dependents) pay(s) some (or all) of the premium for exchange coverage.

Under scenario B, the amount that a taxpayer who receives a premium credit would be required to contribute towards the premium is capped as a percent of household income; that is, the *required premium contribution* would be the product of the taxpayer's household income and the "applicable percentage." In general, the applicable percentage will be less for those with lower incomes compared with those with higher incomes; where income is measured relative to the federal poverty level.

Under scenario B, the amount that taxpayers with income between 100% FPL and 133% FPL will be required to contribute towards the premium will be capped at 2 percent of household income. For taxpayers with income 300%-400% FPL, their premium contribution will be capped at 9.5% of income. ACA further specifies the applicable percentages that premium credit recipients, whose incomes are between those two income bands, would be required to pay towards the cost of exchange coverage under scenario B (see **Figure 2**).

Figure 2. Maximum Percentage of Income, as Measured by FPL, to go towards Premium Contributions

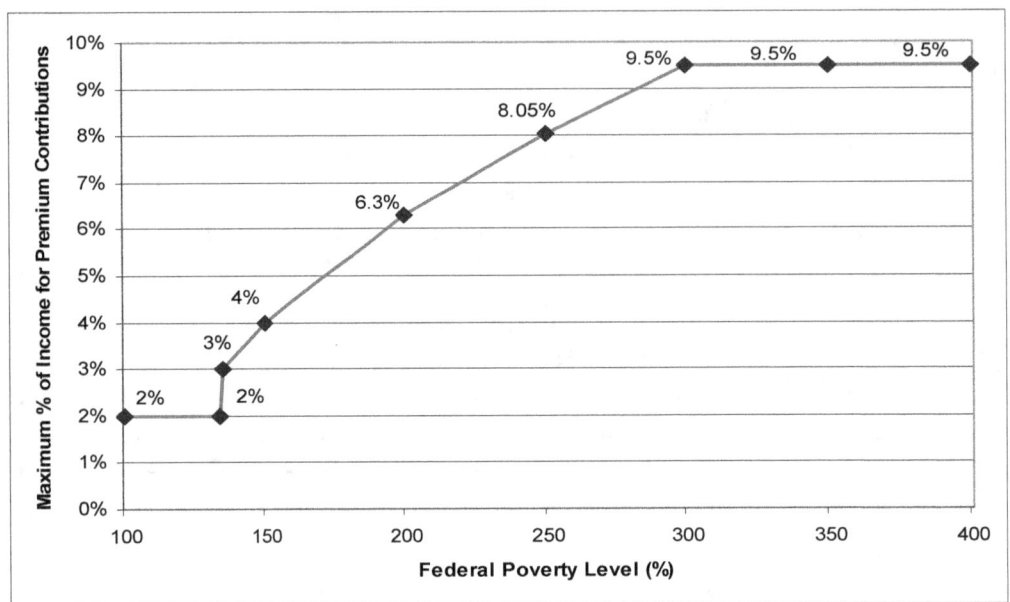

Source: CRS analysis of ACA.

Note: Beginning in 2014, citizens and qualifying legal residents with household income at or below 133% FPL will be e igible for Medicaid rather than premium credits.

Calculation of the *premium credit amount* (under scenario B) would be the arithmetic difference (if any) after subtracting the taxpayer's required premium contribution from the premium for the second lowest cost silver plan ("reference plan") available to the taxpayer. It is *theoretically* possible that a taxpayer's premium contribution could be equal to or exceed the premium for the reference plan, leaving that taxpayer with a premium credit amount of zero. Moreover, premium credit recipients who enroll in plans that are more expensive than the reference plan would have to pay the additional premium amount.

Illustrative Examples: If Premium Credits Were Available in 2011

For illustrative purposes only, if the premium credits were available in 2011, **Table 2** shows annual income levels as measured against the 2011 FPL, by family size.

Table 2. Annual Income by 2011 Federal Poverty Level and Family Size

For the 48 contiguous states and the District of Columbia

Federal Poverty Line (FPL)	Family Size			
	1	2	3	4
0%	$0	$0	$0	$0
50%	$5,445	$7,355	$9,265	$11,175
100%	$10,890	$14,710	$18,530	$22,350
133%	$14,484	$19,564	$24,645	$29,726
150%	$16,335	$22,065	$27,795	$33,525
200%	$21,780	$29,420	$37,060	$44,700
250%	$27,225	$36,775	$46,325	$55,875
300%	$32,670	$44,130	$55,590	$67,050
350%	$38,115	$51,485	$64,855	$78,225
400%	$43,560	$58,840	$74,120	$89,400

Source: CRS computation based on "Annual Update of the HHS Poverty Guide ines," 76 Federal Register 3637-3638, January 20, 2011, http://aspe.hhs.gov/poverty/11fedreg.pdf.

Notes: Under ACA, premium credits for eligible exchange coverage will not be available until 2014; the data in this table are for illustrative purposes only. Different income levels, as measured against the FPL, apply separately to Alaska and Hawaii (see "Annual Update of the HHS Poverty Guidelines" referenced under Source). The Federal Poverty Guidelines are updated annually for inflation.

Also for illustrative purposes, **Table 3** displays the maximum *monthly* amounts that premium credit recipients would be required to contribute towards exchange coverage (provided that they enrolled in the reference plan or a less expensive exchange plan).

Table 3. Maximum Monthly Premium Contributions, by Family Size, If Premium Credits were Available in 2011

(for the 48 contiguous states and the District of Columbia)

Federal Poverty Line (FPL)	Maximum Premium Contribution as a % of Income ("Applicable Percentages")	Maximum Monthly Premium Contribution (2011), by Family Size			
		1	2	3	4
100%	2.0%	$18	$25	$31	$37
133.00%	2.0%	$24	$33	$41	$50
133.01%	3.0%	$36	$49	$62	$74
150%	4.0%	$54	$74	$93	$112
200%	6.3%	$114	$154	$195	$235
250%	8.05%	$183	$247	$311	$375
300%	9.5%	$259	$349	$440	$531
350%	9.5%	$302	$408	$513	$619
400%	9.5%	$345	$466	$587	$708

Source: CRS computation based on "Annual Update of the HHS Poverty Guide ines," 76 Federal Register 3637-3638, January 20, 2011, and ACA.

Notes: Under ACA, premium credits for eligible exchange coverage will not be available until 2014; the data in this table are for illustrative purposes only. Different income levels, as measured against the FPL, apply separately to Alaska and Hawaii (see "Annual Update of the HHS Poverty Guidelines" referenced under Source). The Federal Poverty Guidelines are updated annually for inflation. If individuals enroll in more expensive plans than the second lowest-cost silver plan in their respective areas, they would be responsible for the additional premium amounts. The premium contribution amounts are rounded to the nearest dollar.

Both **Figure 2** and **Table 3** illustrate the "cliff effect" that occurs at 133% FPL. For those at or below 133% FPL who are not eligible for Medicaid but eligible for premium credits (e.g., certain legal permanent residents), the credits will ensure that such individuals pay no more than 2% of their income (if any) for exchange coverage. Above 133% FPL, a formula is applied so that a family at 133.01% FPL will pay 3% of their income for those premiums. For example, as shown in **Table 3**, a family of four with income at 133% FPL ($29,726 in annual income) may be required to pay $50 in monthly premiums, if the exchange and premium credit provisions were currently in effect. With one additional dollar of income ($29,727 in annual income), they would be required to pay $74 in monthly premiums. Thus, in this example, that additional $1 in income would lead to $24 more in required premium payments for the family per month (an additional $288 in premium contributions for the year). Some might observe that prior to the implementation of the ACA premium credits in 2014, an even larger cliff exists for citizens and qualified aliens, whose extra dollar of income makes them ineligible for Medicaid, at which point *no* premium credits were available.

Examples of Premium Credits for Self-Only and Family Coverage

For illustrative purposes, assume that premium credits were available in 2011. The following examples were calculated using the formula specified in ACA (see **Table 4**).[26] The examples assume that the individual or family is/are enrolled in an exchange plan with a premium that exceeds the amount of the premium credit they would receive, and therefore the credit would be based on the reference plan in the local area.

Note that the premium credit amounts are greater for those at the lower end of the eligible income range. The credit amount goes to zero when income is at 400% FPL.

Table 4. Annual Premium Contributions and Annual Premium Credit Amounts, if Credits were Available in 2011, by Coverage Tier

Coverage Tiers	Federal Poverty Level (FPL)	Income Levels based on FPL	Maximum Premium Contribution as a % of Income	Annual Premium	Required Annual Contribution	Annual Credit Amount
Self-Only	100%ᵃ	$10,890	2.0%	$5,000	$218	$4,782
	200%	$21,780	6.3%	$5,000	$1,372	$3,628
	350%	$38,115	9.5%	$5,000	$3,621	$1,379
	400%	N/A	N/A	N/A	N/A	$0
Family of Four	100%	$22,350	2.0%	$13,500	$447	$13,053
	200%	$44,700	6.3%	$13,500	$2,816	$10,684
	350%	$78,225	9.5%	$13,500	$7,431	$6,069
	400%	N/A	N/A	N/A	N/A	$0

Source: CRS computation based on "Annual Update of the HHS Poverty Guide ines," 76 *Federal Register* 3637-3638, January 20, 2011; KFF/HRET, "Employer Health Benefits 2011 Annual Survey," 2011; and ACA.

Notes: Under ACA, premium credits for eligible exchange coverage will not be available until 2014; the data in this table are for illustrative purposes only. Different income levels, as measured against the FPL, apply separately to Alaska and Hawaii (see "Annual Update of the HHS Poverty Guidelines" referenced under Source). The Federal Poverty Guidelines are updated annually for inflation.

a. Most individuals/families with income between 100% and 133% FPL will qualify for Medicaid. However, certain individuals will not: certain legal permanent residents (LPRs) who have resided in the U.S. *less* than five years. For purposes of the premium credit calculation, the income of credit-eligible LPRs will be assumed to be equivalent to 100% FPL.

Self-Only Coverage Examples

Assume that the annual premium for the reference plan (second lowest-cost silver plan) is $5,000 for self-only coverage (see **Table 4**). An individual with income at 200% FPL ($21,780 for 2011),

---

[26] See the text box "Calculations of Premium Credit Amount" for the premium credit formula.

would have a required annual contribution of $1,372 (i.e., $21,780 annual income multiplied by 6.3%). This individual would receive a tax credit of $3,628 for that year (i.e., $5,000 annual premium minus $1,372 required annual contribution), provided that the individual enrolled in an exchange plan with an annual premium that exceeds the credit amount.[27]

Assuming the same $5,000 annual premium for self-only coverage, an individual with income at 350% FPL would be required to contribute $3,621, resulting in a premium credit of $1,379.

Family Coverage Examples

The examples discussed above for self-only coverage may be replicated for purposes of estimating contributions and credit amounts for family coverage. Assume the annual premium for the second lowest-cost silver plan is $13,500 for family coverage (see **Table 4**). A family of four with income at 200% FPL ($44,700 for 2011), would have a required annual contribution of $2,816 (i.e., $44,700 multiplied by 6.3%). This family would receive a tax credit of $10,684 for that year (i.e., $13,500 minus $2,816).

Assuming the same $13,500 annual premium for family coverage, a family of four with income at 350% FPL would be required to contribute $7,431, resulting in a premium credit of $6,069.

Reconciliation of Premium Credits

Under ACA, the amount received in premium credits is based on the prior year's income tax returns. These amounts are reconciled in the next year when individuals file a tax return for the actual year in which they received a premium credit. If a tax filing unit's income changes, and the filer should have received a higher amount, this additional credit would be included in their tax refund for the year. On the other hand, any excess amount that was overpaid in premium credits would have to be repaid to the federal government as a tax payment. However, ACA imposed a limitation on the excess amount repaid for certain households. Specifically, for households with incomes below 400% of the FPL, the amount of repayment cannot exceed $400 (joint filers) and $250 (single filers). This amount will be indexed by inflation in future years.

Since the enactment of ACA, these limits have been increased in order to raise revenues for other legislative initiatives. On December 15, 2010, the Medicare and Medicaid Extenders Act of 2010 (P.L. 111-309) froze Medicare payments for physicians at 2010 rates (instead of the substantial, scheduled payment reduction).[28] The law also included several technical changes to extend existing programs that were scheduled to expire at the end of the year. To offset the cost from these changes, the bill changed the repayment limit for overpayment of premium credits to vary by income class (see **Table 4**).

---

[27] According to ACA's premium credit provisions, in order for the credit amount to be based on the reference plan, the estimated credit amount must exceed the cost of the exchange plan in which the individual/family is enrolled.

[28] See CRS Report R40907, *Medicare Physician Payment Updates and the Sustainable Growth Rate (SGR) System*, by Jim Hahn and Janemarie Mulvey.

Table 5. Limits on Repayment of Excess Premium Credits Enacted by the Medicare and Medicaid Extenders Act (P.L. 111-309)

If the Household Income (Expressed as a Percentage of Poverty Line) Is:	The Applicable Dollar Limit for Joint Filers Is:
Less than 200%	$600
At least 200% but less than 250%	$1,000
At least 250% but less than 300%	$1,500
At least 300% but less than 350%	$2,000
At least 350% but less than 400%	$2,500
At least 400% but less than 450%	$3,000
At least 450% but less than 500%	$3,500

Note: The applicable dollar imit for single filers is 50% of the joint filer limit.

On April 14, 2011, the Comprehensive 1099 Taxpayer Protection and Repayment of Exchange Subsidy Overpayment Act of 2011 (P.L. 112-9) was passed. The law repealed provisions in ACA that expanded the income reporting requirements to certain businesses.[29] To raise revenues to pay for these changes, the law lowered the maximum applicable limits for repayment of excess amount paid in premium credits to those shown in **Table 6**. In addition, those with household income of more than 400% of the FPL and up to 500% of FPL (at the time they filed their tax returns) were no longer subject to caps on repayment of overpayment amounts.

Table 6. Limits on Repayment of Excess Premium Credits Enacted by the Comprehensive 1099 Taxpayer Protection and Repayment of Exchange Subsidy Overpayment Act of 2011 (P.L. 112-9)

If the Household Income (Expressed as a Percentage of Poverty Line) Is:	The Applicable Dollar Limit for Married Filers Is:
Less than 200%	$600
At least 200% but less than 300%	$1,500
At least 300% but less than 400%	$2,500

Note: The applicable dollar imit for single filers is 50% of the joint filer imit.

Most recently, on June 7, 2012, the House passed H.R. 436, the Health Care Cost Reduction Act of 2012, which would repeal an ACA provision that imposed a 2.3% excise tax on manufacturers and importers of a broad range of medical devices. H.R. 436 would also loosen some of the current restrictions on health flexible spending accounts.[30] To raise revenues for these provisions, H.R. 436 includes a measure that would remove all limits on repayment of overpayments of the premium credit, making individuals fully liable for the full amount of any overpayment.

---

[29] See CRS Report R41782, *1099 Information Reporting Requirements and Penalties Recent Legislative Activity*, by Carol A. Pettit and Edward C. Liu

[30] See CRS Report RL32656, *Health Care Flexible Spending Accounts*, by Janemarie Mulvey for more information.

According to the CBO, this change will raise $31.9 billion in revenues over 10 years (2013-2022).[31] The bill will now be sent to the Senate for consideration.

---

[31] Congressional Budget Office, Cost Estimate for the Honorable David Dreier, Chairman, Committee on Rules, June 5, 2012.

Appendix. Health Insurance "Affordability" in the Exchange

While there is no widely accepted definition of individual "affordability" when it comes to health insurance premiums, and other health-care related out-of-pocket costs,[32] ACA sets insurance premium credits for persons, and their covered dependents, such that individuals and families will be required to spend no more than a specified percentage of income on premiums for specified health insurance plans in an exchange. Insurance premium credits under ACA will extend to individuals and families with modified adjusted gross income (hereinafter referred to simply as "income" with respect to ACA) between 100% and 400% FPL. ACA will provide premium credit support scaled to individual and family income relative to poverty such that eligible families' and individuals' premium contributions will be limited from 2.0% to 9.5% of income. Individuals and families with income at or above 400% of poverty will be ineligible for premium credits.

In terms of the premiums, ACA implicitly sets a pre-tax "affordability cap" of 9.5% of income on base coverage plans in the exchange (i.e., plans with a beginning actuarial value of 70%, not including the impact of cost-sharing subsidies), for individuals and families with income up to 400% of poverty.

This section examines only the relative "affordability" of enrollee premiums in health insurance exchanges as a percentage of enrollee's income (adjusted gross income or AGI),[33] considering illustrative plan premiums, after subsidies and, if applicable, any federal tax deduction due to excess medical (i.e., qualifying health insurance and health care) expenses.

The insurance premiums used in the examples are for purposes of illustration only. Ultimately, the premiums individuals would face in the health insurance exchanges will depend on a host of factors, including the varying prices paid by plans for medical goods and services, the breadth of the provider network, the provisions regarding how out-of-network care is paid for (or not), the use of tools by the plan to reduce health care utilization (e.g., prior authorization for certain tests), and other factors. The estimates shown here are based on illustrative premiums developed by the Kaiser Family Foundation (KFF) in 2009.[34] The illustrated plans are estimated to have a 70% actuarial value, meaning that the plans are expected to cover 70% of plan members' covered health care costs, with members' spending on cost-sharing (e.g., deductibles and copayments)

---

[32] ACA includes provisions to study affordability issues. It requires GAO to conduct a survey of the cost and affordability of health care insurance provided under the exchanges for owners and employees of small business concerns, including data on enrollees in exchanges and individuals purchasing health insurance coverage outside of exchanges. GAO is also required to conduct a study on the affordability of health insurance coverage (including the impact of credits for individuals and small businesses), the availability of affordable health benefits plans (including a study of whether the percentage of household income used for credit purposes is appropriate for determining whether employer-provided coverage is affordable and whether such level may be lowered without significantly increasing the costs to the federal government and reducing employer-provided coverage), and the ability of individuals to maintain essential health benefits coverage. ACA also requires the HHS Secretary to conduct a study examining the feasibility and implication of adjusting the FPL for premium and cost-sharing credits for different geographic areas so as to reflect the variations in cost-of-living among different areas. If the Secretary determines that an adjustment is feasible, the study should include a methodology to make such an adjustment.

[33] While the definition of income for the purposes of premium credit eligibility uses MAGI, for ease of analysis the illustrations discussed in this section uses AGI as the definition of income.

[34] http://healthreform.kff.org/SubsidyCalculator.aspx, accessed on March 23, 2010.

---

covering the remaining 30%. In the exchanges, insurers will be allowed to age-rate premiums within prescribed bands—under ACA, the highest age-adjusted premium can be no more than three times the lowest age-adjusted premium. ACA also will allow premiums to vary by tobacco use (by no more than 1.5:1 ratio) and geographic area.

Figure A-1 depicts the relative "affordability" of health insurance premiums prior to the application of the credits and ACA as of 2014, depicting out-of-pocket premiums as a percentage of income. The figure is based on KFF's illustrated health insurance plan cost of $5,428 for a 50-year-old with single coverage living in a medium-cost area. Out-of-pocket premiums are shown based on pre-tax as well as post-tax premiums, using the excess medical expense threshold limit of 7.5% of adjusted gross income prior to ACA, and 10.0% after ACA.

The figure shows that at 100% of poverty, the illustrated insurance plan would cost individuals *half* of their pre-tax income prior to ACA—insurance premiums at this level, amounting to 50% of pre-tax income, would be considered unaffordable by many, and could crowd out spending on other basic needs such as food, shelter and utilities, and clothing. Prior to ACA, the 7.5% excess medical expense deduction was the only federal subsidy toward the cost of their medical insurance that these individuals were eligible to receive; at lower-income levels the deduction had little or no effect on net post-tax premiums. Under ACA, Medicaid will be expanded to 133% FPL, which will permit individuals to enroll with relatively limited or no premiums and cost-sharing. Under the depicted plan, health insurance premiums after reflecting ACA's subsidies would range from 3% of income at just above 133% of poverty, up to 9.5% of income at just under 400% FPL. At 400% FPL, individuals are shown bearing the full pre-tax cost of the illustrated plan ($5,428), which would amount to 12.5% of their pre-tax income; after applying the excess medical expense deduction under current law, the post-tax premium amounts to 11.7% of adjusted gross (pre-tax) income.

Figure A-1. ACA Compared to Pre-ACA Premiums:
Pre- and Post-tax Out-of-Pocket Premiums
as a Percentage of Adjusted Gross Income

Based on Illustrated Annual Insurance Plan Cost for a 50-Year-Old with Single Coverage
in a Medium-Cost Area ($5,428)

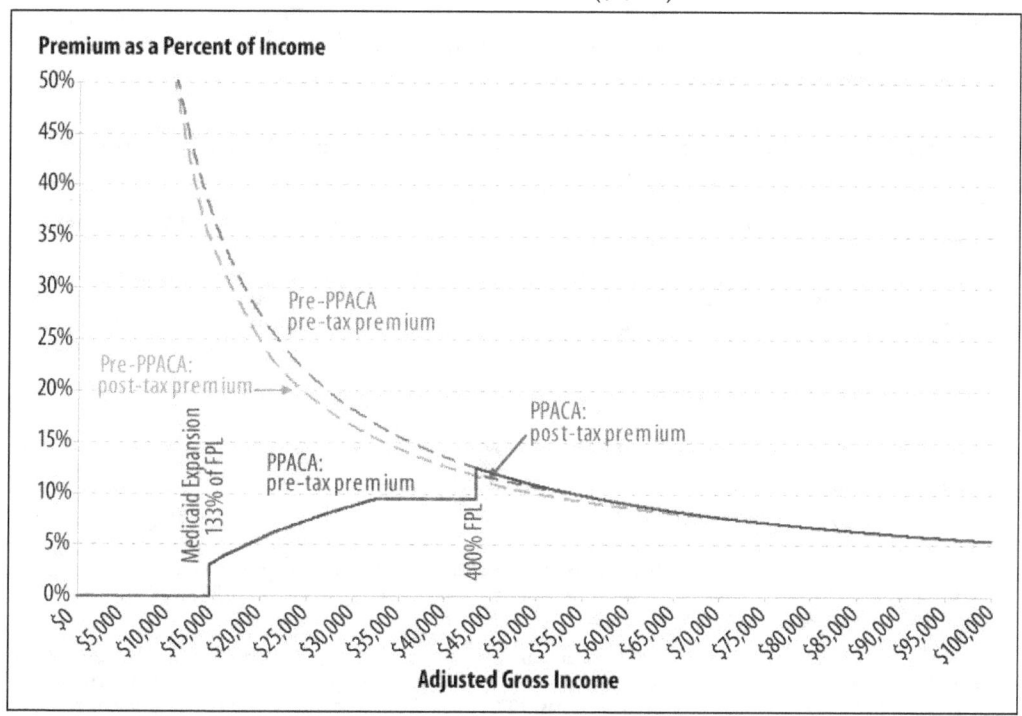

Source: Prepared by CRS based on Kaiser Family Foundation (KFF) illustrative health insurance premiums, for plans with an estimated actuarial value of 70%, in 2009.

Notes: Estimates are for illustration only, based on illustrated KFF health insurance premiums. Actual premiums would ikely vary among health insurance exchanges based on a wide range of factors. The figure shows that prior to ACA, no premium credits are provided to individuals under 400% FPL, with the only federal subsidy being the effect of the deduction of medical expenses in excess of the 7.5% AGI threshold (as illustrated by the post-tax premium). ACA provides premium credits up to 400% of FPL, but increases the excess medical expense deduction threshold to 10.0% of AGI.

Illustrated Potential Effects of Age-Banding and Area Cost Adjustments on "Affordability"

Table A-1 shows illustrative KFF plan premiums in the exchange based on 2009 plan costs.[35] The examples shown here reflect the possible effects of age-banding of premiums and geographic cost variation on health insurance premium affordability. In the examples shown, KFF illustrative premiums in higher-cost areas are set at 20% above those in medium-cost areas, and premiums in

---

[35] Given that KFF developed their illustrative premiums in 2009, the original analysis compared such amounts to the federal poverty levels applicable for that year. Since FPLs are adjusted annually, the FPLs used in the analysis in the Appendix of the paper are different from the FPLs used elsewhere in the report.

lower-cost areas are set 20% below. Under KFF's age-banding, premiums for 30-year-olds are only slightly above those of 20-year-olds. At age 40, premiums are one-third higher than at age 20; at age 50, just over twice; and at age 60, three times as high (consistent with the age-banding limits). KFF estimates single+1 premiums as simply twice those of single coverage. Premiums for a family of four follow a similar age progression, except at age 50, premiums are only 84% higher than for 20-year-olds, and for 60-year-olds, 1.6 times higher.[36] Further discussion will focus on single individuals and couples (married and unmarried) under single premium and single+1 premium plans.

Table A-1. ACA: Illustrative Health Insurance Premiums, by Enrollee Age, Geographic Cost, and Plan Type, 2009

	Single premium			Single+1 premium			Family of four premium		
Age	Lower-cost area	Medium-cost area	Higher-cost area	Lower-cost area	Medium-cost area	Higher-cost area	Lower-cost area	Medium-cost area	Higher-cost area
20	$2,110	$2,637	$3,165	$4,220	$5,274	$6,330	$5,687	$7,108	$8,530
30	$2,141	$2,676	$3,211	$4,282	$5,352	$6,422	$6,290	$7,862	$9,435
40	$2,800	$3,500	$4,200	$5,600	$7,000	$8,400	$7,548	$9,435	$11,321
50	$4,342	$5,428	$6,513	$8,684	$10,856	$13,026	$10,489	$13,112	$15,734
60	$6,329	$7,911	$9,494	$12,658	$15,822	$18,988	$14,960	$18,700	$22,440

Source: Prepared by CRS from Kaiser Family Foundation (KFF) illustrative health insurance premiums, for plans with an estimated actuarial value of 70%, in 2009. Available online at http://healthreform.kff.org/SubsidyCalculator.aspx, accessed on March 23, 2010.

Note: Estimates are for illustration only. Illustrated premiums reflect a 3:1 age-banding, with premiums of oldest enrollees being three times those of youngest enrollees. Illustrated premiums in lower-cost areas are 20% lower than in medium-cost areas, and in higher-cost areas, 20% higher. Actual premiums will likely vary among health insurance exchanges based on a wide range of factors.

Table A-2. ACA: Illustrative Health Insurance Premiums as a Percentage of Income at an Income Level of 400% of the Federal Poverty Level, by Enrollee Age, Geographic Cost, and Plan Type, 2009

	Single premium[a]			Single+1 premium[b]			Family of four premium[c]		
Age	Lower-cost area	Medium-cost area	Higher-cost area	Lower-cost area	Medium-cost area	Higher-cost area	Lower-cost area	Medium-cost area	Higher-cost area
20	4.9%	6.1%	7.3%	7.2%	9.0%	10.9%	6.4%	8.1%	9.7%
30	4.9%	6.2%	7.4%	7.3%	9.2%	11.0%	7.1%	8.9%	10.7%
40	6.5%	8.1%	9.7%	9.6%	12.0%	14.4%	8.6%	10.7%	12.8%
50	10.0%	12.5%	15.0%	14.9%	18.6%	22.4%	11.9%	14.9%	17.8%

---

[36] Presumably the smaller difference for family coverage by age, compared to single coverage, is due to an assumption that by age 50, couples' children tend to be older than those of younger couples, and older children generally have lower health care utilization rates than younger children.

	Single premium[a]			Single+1 premium[b]			Family of four premium[c]		
Age	Lower-cost area	Medium-cost area	Higher-cost area	Lower-cost area	Medium-cost area	Higher-cost area	Lower-cost area	Medium-cost area	Higher-cost area
60	*14.6%*	*18.3%*	*21.9%*	*21.7%*	*27.1%*	*32.6%*	*17.0%*	*21.2%*	*25.4%*

Source: Prepared by CRS based on Kaiser Family Foundation (KFF) illustrative health insurance premiums, for plans with an estimated actuarial value of 70%, in 2009. Available online at http://healthreform.kff.org/ SubsidyCalculator.aspx, accessed on March 23, 2010.

Note: Estimates are for illustration only, based on illustrated KFF health insurance premiums. Actual premiums will likely vary among health insurance exchanges based on a wide range of factors. Values in **bold italic** are above ACA's premium cap of 9.5% of income, extending up to 400% of FPL.

a. Premium as a percentage of income based on 400% of FPL for a single person ($43,320).

b. Premium as a percentage of income based on 400% of FPL for a 2-person family ($58,280).

c. Premium as a percentage of income based on 400% of FPL for a 4-person family ($88,200).

Table A-2 shows the illustrative KFF plan premiums as a percentage of income at 400% of the FPL, the point at which an individual or family no longer is eligible for premium subsidies under ACA. The table shows, for example, that 20- to 40-year-olds in the illustrated single plans have premiums ranging from 4.9% of income (for the youngest group in lower-cost areas), up to 8.1% for 40-year-olds in medium-cost areas—all below the ACA's implicit 9.5% affordability limit. For 40-year-olds in higher-cost areas, illustrated premiums (9.7% of income) are slightly above the law's affordability limit. For 50- and 60-year-olds, the illustrated premiums are above the 9.5% affordability limit in all markets, ranging from 10.0% to 15.0% of income for 50-year-olds, and 14.6% to 21.9% of income for 60-year-olds.[37]

Figure A-2 through **Figure A-4** depict pre- and post-tax premiums as a percentage of income under illustrated self-coverage plans, by enrollee age, in lower-cost, medium-cost, and higher-cost areas, respectively. **Figure A-2**, for example, shows that under the illustrated premiums for a lower-cost area all enrollees with incomes below 400% of poverty would have pre-tax premiums amounting to less than 9.5% income—ACA's affordability cap—due to the law's premium credits. However, the impact of age-rating premiums will differ for younger vs. older individuals, as their income increases. For example, for individuals age 30 and 40, the illustrated premiums as a percentage of income naturally decline before reaching the 400% FPL, because they face relatively low premiums (compared with older individuals) as their income increases. In contrast, individuals age 40 and 50 face higher exchange premiums and benefit from the 9.5% income affordability cap all the way up to the 400% income-eligibility limit. At 400% of poverty, illustrated premiums for the 50-year-olds increase slightly, to 10.0% of income, and for 60-year-olds, more substantially, to 14.6% of income.

In medium-cost areas, illustrated in **Figure A-3**, pre-tax premiums for 50-year-olds amount to 12.5% of income, and for 60-year-olds, 18.3% at 400% of the FPL. In higher-cost areas, illustrated in **Figure A-4**, pre-tax premiums at 400% of poverty amount to 15% of income for 50-

---

[37] One study found that annual premiums in the nongroup market for 60- to 64-year-olds averaged $5,755 in 2009, which would be 13.3% of income for an individual at 400% FPL. See Table 2, "Individual Health Insurance," AHIP Center for Policy and Research, October 2009.

year-olds, and 21.9% of income for 60-year-olds. For 60-year-olds, pre-tax premiums fall back to 9.5% of income once income reaches $99,937 or 923% FPL.

Figure A-5 through **Figure A-7** depict pre- and post-tax premiums as a percentage of income under illustrated plans, for a married couple with no children having "single+1" insurance coverage, by enrollee age, in three geographic cost areas. The illustrated premiums for "single+1" coverage are twice those for single coverage. **Table A-2** shows that for a married couple with a single+1 policy, at 400% of poverty, illustrated premiums in lower-cost areas for 50- and 60-year-olds are well above the 9.5% "affordability threshold" with illustrated premiums at 14.9% of income for 50-year-olds, and 21.7% for 60-year-olds. In medium-cost areas, illustrated premiums at 400% of poverty for a 40-year-old (12.0% of income) are above the 9.5% "affordability threshold," and range up to 27.1% of income for 60-year-olds. For married-couples in higher-cost areas, illustrated premiums at 400% of poverty are higher than the 9.5% "affordability threshold" at all ages, ranging from 10.9% of income for a 20-year-old, up to 32.6% for 60-year-old enrollees.

It should be noted that the figures that follow reflect estimates under ACA only, unlike **Figure A-1**, which illustrates pre- and post-tax premiums both before and after ACA.

Figure A-2. ACA: Pre- and Post-Tax Out-of-Pocket Premiums as a Percentage of Adjusted Gross Income, by Age—Single Policy in a Lower-Cost Area

Based on Illustrated Annual Insurance Plan Costs—
Age 30: $2,141, Age 40: $2,800, Age 50: $4,342, Age 60: $6,329

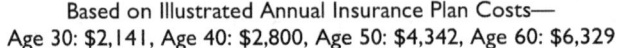
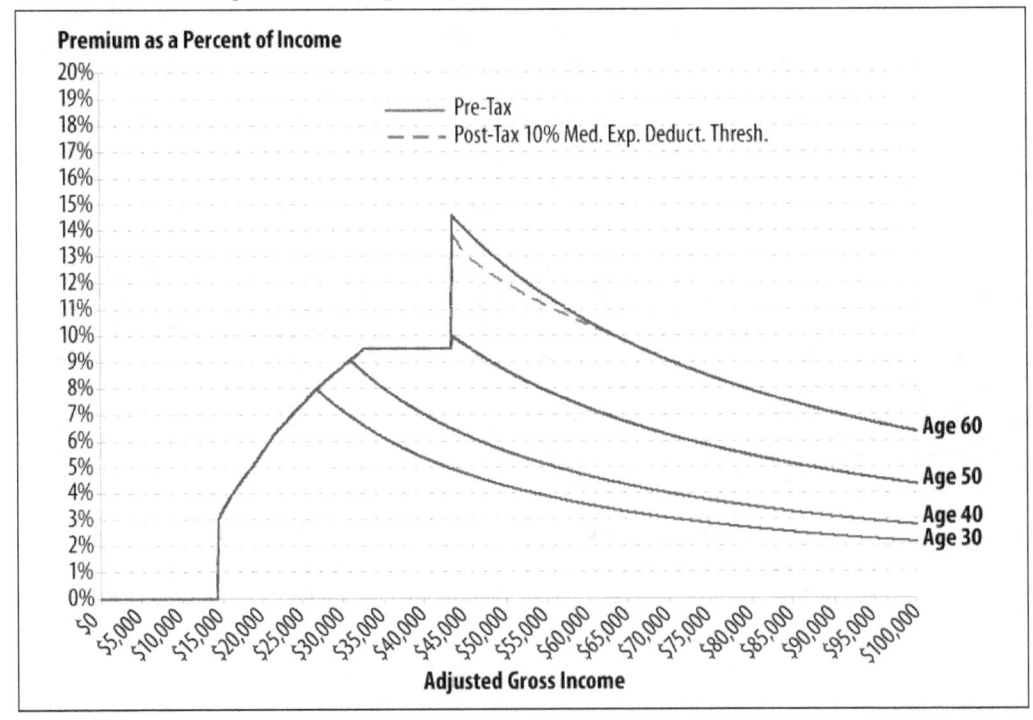

Source: Prepared by CRS based on Kaiser Family Foundation (KFF) illustrative health insurance premiums, for plans with an estimated actuarial value of 70%, in 2009.

Notes: Estimates are for illustration only, based on illustrated KFF health insurance premiums. Actual premiums would ikely vary among health insurance exchanges based on a wide range of factors. Persons and families with incomes of 400% of poverty and above would be ineligible for premium subsidy support, and their pre-tax premiums would be the same they faced prior to ACA (absent other effects the law might have on reducing the price of health insurance). Net post-tax premiums are based ACA's excess medical expense deduction threshold of 10.0%.

Figure A-3. ACA: Pre- and Post-Tax Out-of-Pocket Premiums as a Percentage of Adjusted Gross Income, by Age—Single Policy in a Medium-Cost Area

Based on Illustrated Annual Insurance Plan Costs—

Age 30: $2,676, Age 40: $3,500, Age 50: $5,428, Age 60: $7,911

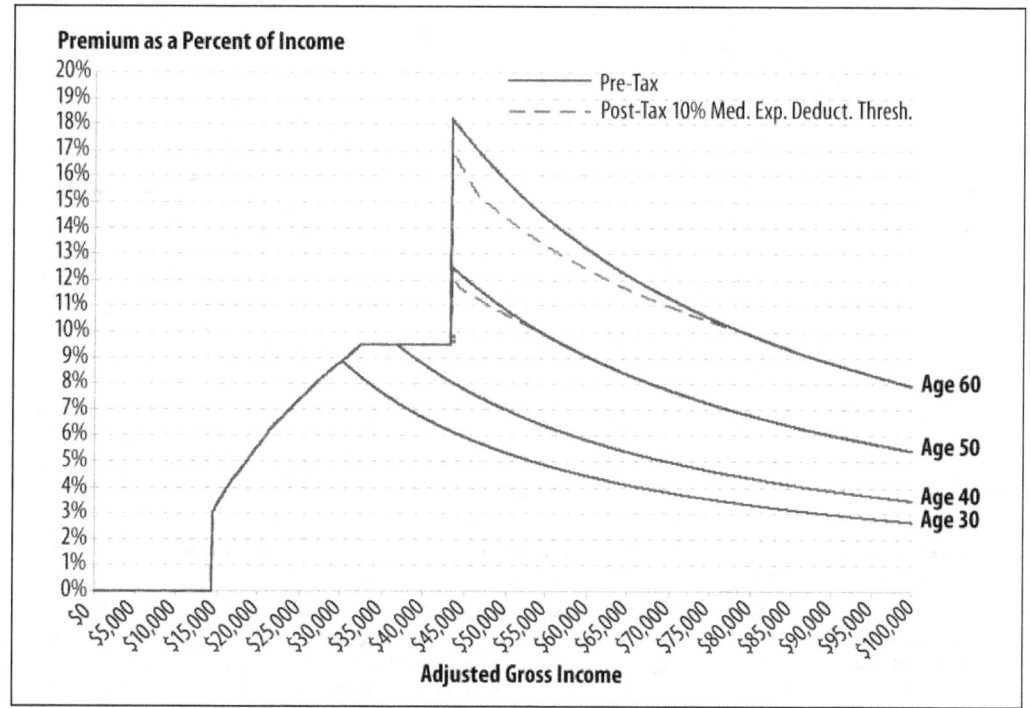

Source: Prepared by CRS based on Kaiser Family Foundation (KFF) illustrative health insurance premiums, for plans with an estimated actuarial value of 70%, in 2009.

Notes: Estimates are for illustration only, based on illustrated KFF health insurance premiums. Actual premiums would ikely vary among health insurance exchanges based on a wide range of factors. Persons and families with incomes of 400% of poverty and above would be ineligible for premium subsidy support, and their pre-tax premiums would be the same they faced prior to ACA (absent other effects the law might have on reducing the price of health insurance). Net post-tax premiums are based ACA's excess medical expense deduction threshold of 10.0%.

Figure A-4. ACA: Pre- and Post-Tax Out-of-Pocket Premiums as a Percentage of Adjusted Gross Income, by Age—Single Policy in a Higher-Cost Area

Based on Illustrative Annual Insurance Plan Costs—

Age 30: $3,211, Age 40: $4,200, Age 50: $6,513, Age 60: $9,494

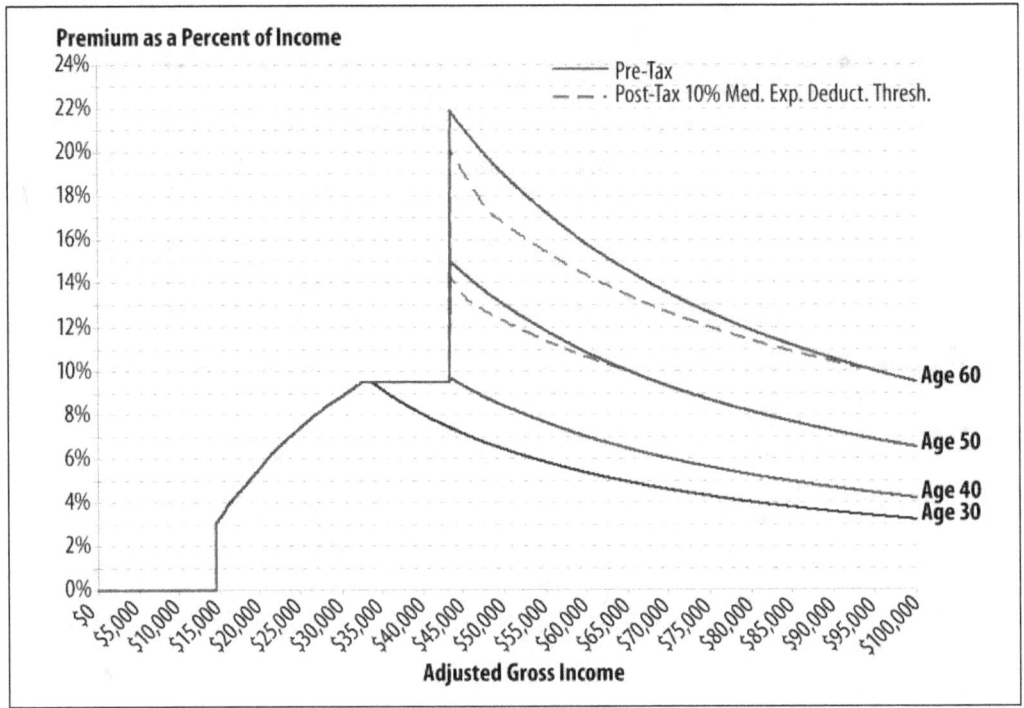

Source: Prepared by CRS based on Kaiser Family Foundation (KFF) illustrative health insurance premiums, for plans with an estimated actuarial value of 70%, in 2009.

Notes: Estimates are for illustration only, based on illustrated KFF health insurance premiums. Actual premiums would ikely vary among health insurance exchanges based on a wide range of factors. Persons and families with incomes of 400% of poverty and above would be ineligible for premium subsidy support, and their pre-tax premiums would be the same they faced prior to ACA (absent other effects the law might have on reducing the price of health insurance). Net post-tax premiums are based ACA's excess medical expense deduction threshold of 10.0%.

**Figure A-5. ACA: Pre- and Post-Tax Out-of-Pocket Premiums as a Percentage of Adjusted Gross Income, by Age—
Married Couple with no Children, Single+1 Policy in a Lower-Cost Area**

Based on Illustrated Annual Insurance Plan Costs—
Age 30: $4,282, Age 40: $5,600, Age 50: $8,684, Age 60: $12,658

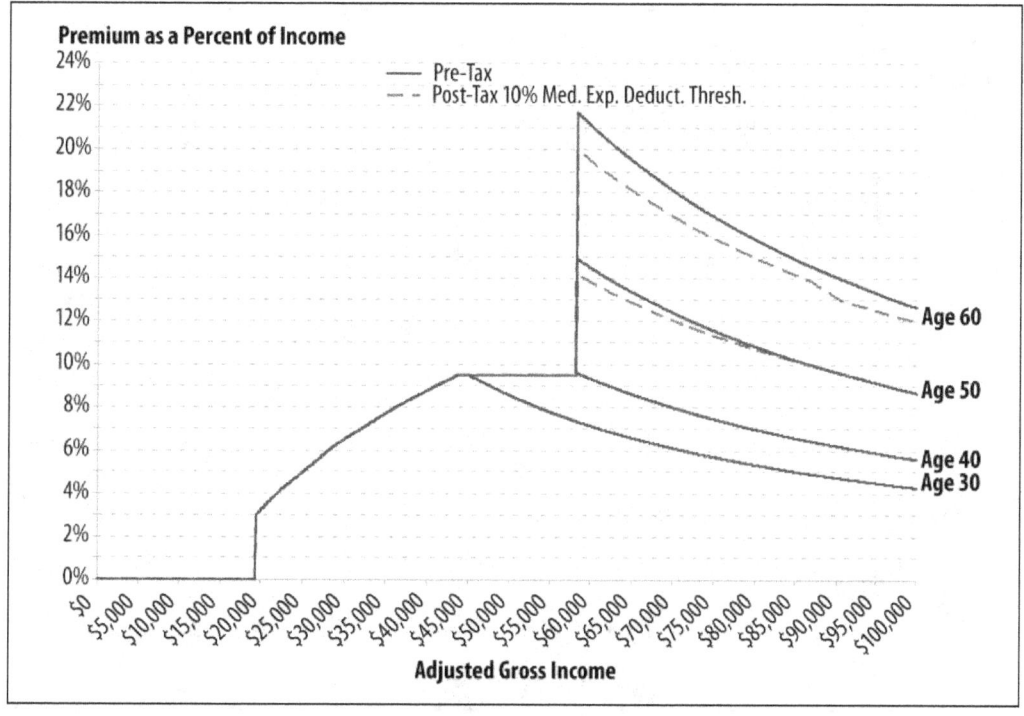

Source: Prepared by CRS based on Kaiser Family Foundation (KFF) illustrative health insurance premiums, for plans with an estimated actuarial value of 70%, in 2009.

Notes: Estimates are for illustration only, based on illustrated KFF health insurance premiums. Actual premiums would likely vary among health insurance exchanges based on a wide range of factors. Persons and families with incomes of 400% of poverty and above would be ineligible for premium subsidy support, and their pre-tax premiums would be the same they faced prior to ACA (absent other effects the law might have on reducing the price of health insurance). Net post-tax premiums are based ACA's excess medical expense deduction threshold of 10.0%.

Figure A-6. ACA: Pre- and Post-Tax Out-of-Pocket Premiums as a Percentage of Adjusted Gross Income, by Age—
Married Couple with no Children, Single+1 Policy in a Medium-Cost Area

Based on Illustrated Annual Insurance Plan Costs—

Age 30: $5,352, Age 40: $7,000, Age 50: $10,856, Age 60: $15,822

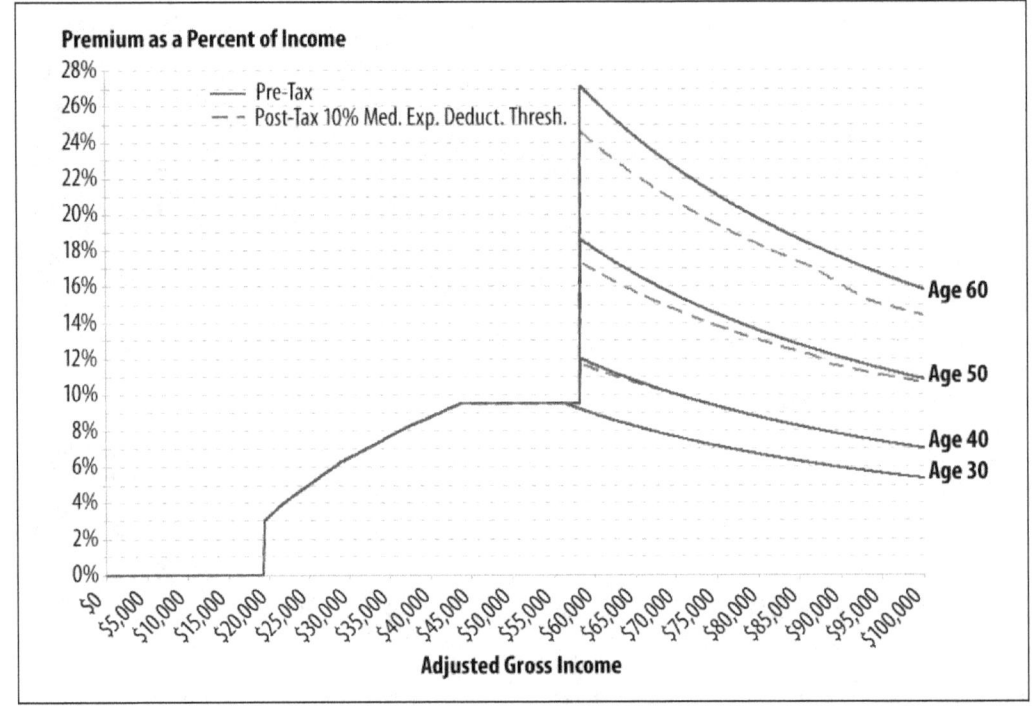

Source: Prepared by CRS based on Kaiser Family Foundation (KFF) illustrative health insurance premiums, for plans with an estimated actuarial value of 70%, in 2009.

Notes: Estimates are for illustration only, based on illustrated KFF health insurance premiums. Actual premiums would ikely vary among health insurance exchanges based on a wide range of factors. Persons and families with incomes of 400% of poverty and above would be ineligible for premium subsidy support, and their pre-tax premiums would be the same they faced prior to ACA (absent other effects the law might have on reducing the price of health insurance). Net post-tax premiums are based ACA's excess medical expense deduction threshold of 10.0%.

Figure A-7. ACA: Pre- and Post-Tax Out-of-Pocket Premiums as a Percentage of Adjusted Gross Income, by Age—
Married Couple with no Children, Single+1 Policy in a Higher-Cost Area

Based on Illustrated Annual Insurance Plan Costs—

Age 30: $6,422, Age 40: $8,400, Age 50: $13,026, Age 60: $18,988

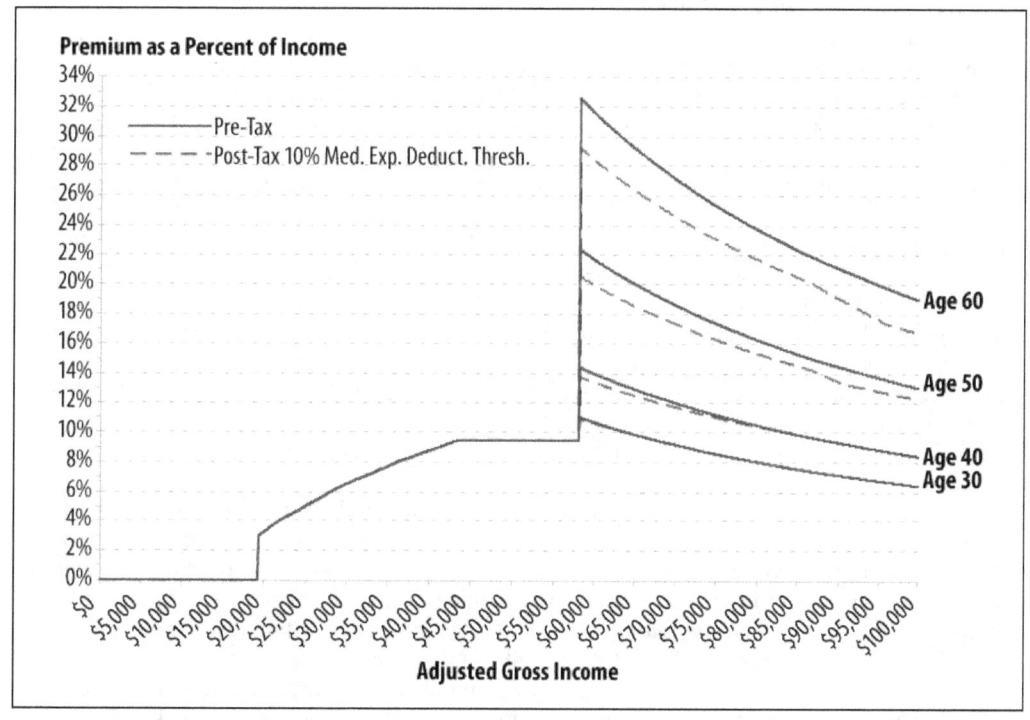

Source: Prepared by CRS based on Kaiser Family Foundation (KFF) illustrative health insurance premiums, for plans with an estimated actuarial value of 70%, in 2009.

Notes: Estimates are for illustration only, based on illustrated KFF health insurance premiums. Actual premiums would ikely vary among health insurance exchanges based on a wide range of factors. Persons and families with incomes of 400% of poverty and above would be ineligible for premium subsidy support, and their pre-tax premiums would be the same they faced prior to ACA (absent other effects the law might have on reducing the price of health insurance). Net post-tax premiums are based ACA's excess medical expense deduction threshold of 10.0%.

Relative "Affordability" of Premiums for Married and Unmarried Couples

Some have described the structure of the premium support provided under ACA's health insurance exchanges, with respect to the phase out of premium support relative to enrollees' income, as resulting in a "marriage penalty."[38] Under ACA's health insurance exchanges, a couple may receive a lesser subsidy, and consequently incur higher out-of-pocket insurance premiums, if

---

[38] Martin Vaughan, "Married Couples Pay More than Unmarried Under Health Bill," *Wall Street Journal*, January 6, 2010, online edition. Available online at http://online.wsj.com/article/SB126281943134818675.html.

they are married, as opposed to unmarried, all other things being equal, thus resulting in a "marriage penalty."[39] ACA phases out premium support on the basis of income relative to the Federal Poverty Level. Premium support in the exchanges for a married couple would be based on their combined income relative to the FPL for two persons ($14,570), and if unmarried, based on their individual incomes relative to the FPL for one person ($10,830). Because the FPL for the married couple is not twice that of a single person, but only 35% higher (i.e., $14,570/$10,830), premium support phases out at a faster rate for the married couple than for the unmarried couple, with equal incomes and combined (pre-subsidy) insurance plan costs. If married, the couple would be ineligible for premium support in the exchange once their income reaches $58,280 (i.e., 400% of the FPL), but if unmarried, premium support could potentially be retained until each individual's income reaches 400% for a single person ($43,320), or potentially until their combined income reaches $86,640 (which would be 595% FPL for a married couple).[40]

The FPL, as originally constructed, recognized that while two persons cannot live as cheaply as one, they can live more cheaply living together, than living apart. In other words, there are economic gains that result from "economies of scale" from living jointly, rather than apart. "Marriage penalties" can result to the extent that FPLs assign lower cost to each additional family member, regardless of whether that family member is a spouse, children, etc.[41] In addition, "marriage penalties" may result more directly from the definition of the economic unit to which the FPL, or other income criteria, is applied.[42] Following are two examples of other federal programs that illustrate how the definition of the economic unit can affect couples' eligibility.

Many federal programs use the FPL as the basis for determining eligibility, setting benefit levels, and phasing out benefits. For example, the Supplemental Nutrition Assistance Program (SNAP) (formerly named the Food Stamp program) counts *household* income for purposes of determining household income eligibility. *Households* with gross income above 100% of poverty are ineligible for the program, as are *households* with net income (after certain disregards) above 130% of poverty. With respect to SNAP, a married couple is treated the same as an unmarried couple, if living together in the same *household*. So, in this context, there is no inherent "marriage penalty" in SNAP, even though it uses the FPL. However, there is a potential "penalty" for two persons living apart, where one or both are receiving SNAP benefits, if they choose to live together, as their combined household income might make them ineligible for SNAP benefits. However, by living together, rather than separately, two individuals, whether married or unmarried, could benefit from implied economies of scale.

In contrast, the Earned Income Tax Credit (EITC) may be said to have a "marriage penalty," even though it does not use the FPL to scale benefits. This is because two unrelated unmarried individuals are treated as individuals under the tax code (single filers), whereas if married their

---

[39] The Treasury Department, in the NPRM on premium credits, requested comments on providing relief to individuals who would receive less premium support after they marry during the tax year. The comment period ended on October 31, 2011. *Federal Register*, Vol. 76, No. 159 , Aug. 17, 2011.

[40] This assumes that the two members of the unmarried couple have individual incomes that are equal. For the married couple, it makes no difference how their income is split.

[41] The 2009 federal poverty levels were $10,830 for an individual, and $3,740 for each additional person.

[42] Because premium credit amounts under the exchanges will be scaled based on income relative to poverty, other types of individuals might find differences in their premiums depending on their living arrangements, other than just whether they're married or not. For example, the total premiums for a single parent with two older children (e.g., age 18 to 25) might differ depending on whether the children enroll separately, based on their individual income, or under the umbrella of a family policy, based on the parent's and children's combined income.

incomes are combined and they are treated as married joint filers. With respect to the EITC, one or both individuals could be eligible for the EITC based on their individual earnings, if unmarried, but become ineligible, or receive a lesser benefit, if they were married, as the EITC would then be based on their combined earnings.

Figure A-8 and **Figure A-9** compare premiums under ACA as a percentage of income for a married couple relative to an unmarried couple, in a medium-cost area, at age 30 and age 50, respectively. The figures show that premiums as a percentage of income would be higher for a married couple than if the couple were unmarried, even though their incomes and insurance premiums are the same.[43]

In the illustrated example at age 30 (**Figure A-8**), the difference in premiums between married and unmarried couples, and as a percentage of income, is much greater, as the married couple's premium subsidy phases out at a faster rate based on its income than it does for the unmarried couple based on their combined income. In the illustration, the married couple no longer receives premium support once their income exceeds $56,337. At that point their premium as a percentage of income naturally falls below ACA's 9.5% "affordability cap," and they are deemed to no longer need premium subsidy support. For the unmarried couple at the same combined income level, assuming their income is equally split, they are individually eligible for premium support of $326 each, based on their individual income ($28,168), and thereby would receive combined premium support of $652. In the example, the unmarried couple's combined premiums amount to 8.3% of their combined income, compared to 9.5% for their married counterpart.

The "marriage penalty" effect increases to the extent premiums exceed the 9.5% "affordability cap" at the point at which a married couple no longer qualifies for premium support (i.e., 400% of poverty, or $58,280). For example, for the 50-year-old couple depicted in **Figure A-9**, at an income level just below $58,280 (i.e., 400% of poverty for the married couple) their premium as a percentage of income is at the 9.5% cap if they are married and 8.6% if they are unmarried. However, the married couple loses premium subsidy support once their income reaches $58,280, and their premium nearly doubles, amounting to 18.6% of their income. In contrast, the unmarried couple continues to be eligible for premium support, at the same combined income level and plan cost as their married counterpart; their combined premiums amount to 8.6% of their combined income—less than half that of the married couple. In the example, both members of the unmarried couple would continue to receive premium support until their individual income reaches $43,320 (400% of the FPL for a single individual), which amounts to a combined income of $86,640. At that, and higher, combined income levels, the unmarried and married couples' premiums are identical, since neither would then qualify for premium credits.

---

[43] For the 30-year-old couple, if they're married, $5,352 for a single+1 policy, and if they're unmarried, each with a $2,676 single policy, amounting to $5,352 combined. For the 50-year-old couple, if they're married, $10,586 for a single+1 policy, and if they're unmarried, each with a $5,428 single policy, amounting to $10,586 combined. The figures assume the two members of the unmarried couple have equal income. Results would differ if their income were split unequally. For the married couple, it makes no difference as to how their income is split.

Figure A-8. ACA: Pre- and Post-Tax Out-of-Pocket Premiums as a Percentage of Adjusted Gross Income, Comparison of Two Couples Age 30 (Married and Unmarried) in a Medium-Cost Area

Based on Illustrative Annual Insurance Plan Costs—
Married Single+1: $5,352, Unmarried Couple: $5,352 ($2,676 Each)

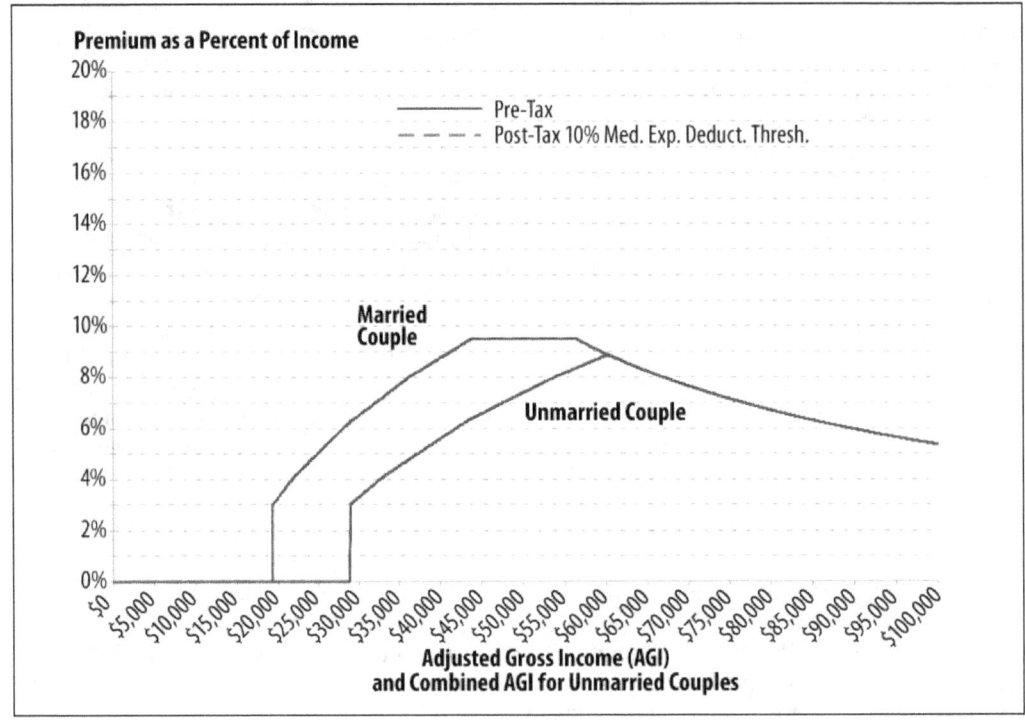

Source: Prepared by CRS based on Kaiser Family Foundation (KFF) illustrative health insurance premiums, for plans with an estimated actuarial value of 70%, in 2009.

Notes: Estimates are for illustration only, based on illustrated KFF health insurance premiums. Actual premiums would ikely vary among health insurance exchanges based on a wide range of factors. Persons and families with incomes of 400% of poverty and above would be ineligible for premium subsidy support, and their pre-tax premiums would be the same they faced prior to ACA (absent other effects the law might have on reducing the price of health insurance). Net post-tax premiums are based ACA's excess medical expense deduction threshold of 10.0%. Under this example, gross premiums are below the 10% excess medical expense deduction threshold at all income levels.

Figure A-9. ACA: Pre- and Post-Tax Out-of-Pocket Premiums as a Percentage of Adjusted Gross Income, Comparison of Two Couples Age 50 (Married and Unmarried) in a Medium-Cost Area

Based on Illustrative Annual Insurance Plan Costs—
Married Single+1: $10,856, Unmarried Couple: $10,856 ($5,428 Each)

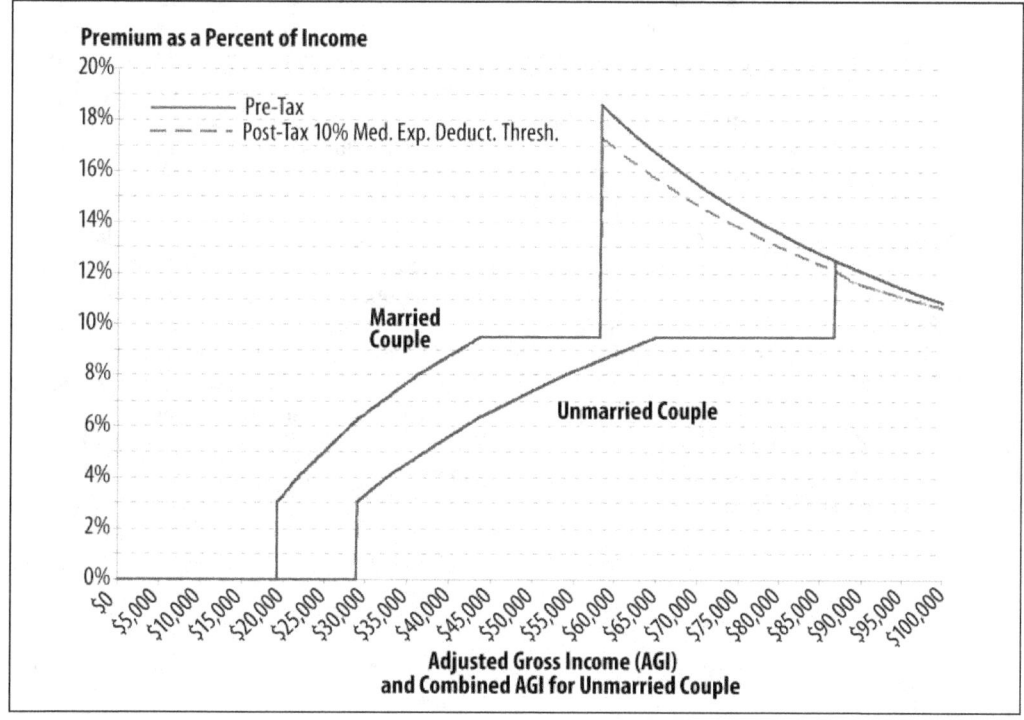

Source: Prepared CRS based on Kaiser Family Foundation (KFF) illustrative health insurance premiums, for plans with an estimated actuarial value of 70%, in 2009.

Notes: Estimates are for illustration only, based on illustrated KFF health insurance premiums. Actual premiums would likely vary among health insurance exchanges based on a wide range of factors. Persons and families with incomes of 400% of poverty and above would be ineligible for premium subsidy support, and their pre-tax premiums would be the same they faced prior to ACA (absent other effects the law might have on reducing the price of health insurance). Net post-tax premiums are based ACA's excess medical expense deduction threshold of 10.0%.

Conclusion

Relative affordability of health insurance premiums individuals and families might face within health insurance exchanges will likely vary from exchange to exchange based on a host of factors. The examples shown in this report are for illustration only, depicting a range by which premiums might reasonably be expected to vary.

ACA will directly improve health insurance affordability for individuals and families with income up to 400% of poverty, by ensuring that no individual or family would pay more than 9.5% of their income for a health insurance plan with an actuarial value of 70% (not including the impact of cost-sharing subsidies). Additionally, ACA will extend Medicaid coverage to 133% of poverty for many individuals, which will permit them to enroll with relatively little or no premiums and cost-sharing. Persons and families with incomes of 400% of poverty and above will be ineligible for premium subsidy support, and their premiums will be the same they would have faced before ACA (absent other effects the law might have on reducing the price of health insurance). Individuals and families who are younger and/or who live in lower-cost areas, as opposed to higher-cost areas, may be able to find plans offered in the exchange costing 9.5% or less of income at some income ranges below 400% of poverty. Others might face exchange premiums that well exceed 9.5% of income, but due to ACA's premium subsidy support their premiums will be capped until their income reaches 400% of poverty. At that point, enrollees might incur abrupt, and in some cases substantial, increases in their health insurance premiums. Additionally, ACA raises the excess medical expense deduction threshold from 7.5% to 10.0% of AGI. Consequently, some individuals and families may find their post-tax insurance premiums to be higher after ACA than before, all other things being equal.

ACA phases out premium support subsidies based on individuals' or families' income relative to poverty. Because the FPL for the married couple is not twice that of a single person, but only 35% higher (i.e., $14,570/$10,830), premium support under ACA phases out at a faster rate relative to *income* for a married couple than it does for a single person, even though the phase-out rate relative to the *FPL* is the same. The structure of the phase-out results in what some might describe as a "marriage penalty." One or both individuals in a couple who are unmarried might be eligible for premium support subsidies based on their individual incomes, but if they married they might not, based on their combined income; if found eligible, the premium subsidy they might receive as a married couple could be less than the combined premium subsidies they might receive as an unmarried couple.

Author Contact Information

Bernadette Fernandez
Specialist in Health Care Financing
bfernandez@crs.loc.gov, 7-0322

Thomas Gabe
Specialist in Social Policy
tgabe@crs.loc.gov, 7-7357

Acknowledgments

The authors wish to thank Chris L. Peterson, former CRS Specialist in Health Care Financing, who co-authored the original report. Janemarie Mulvey authored the section on Reconciliation of Premium Credits.